# Proper Care
# *and* Feeding
# Of Hemorrhoids

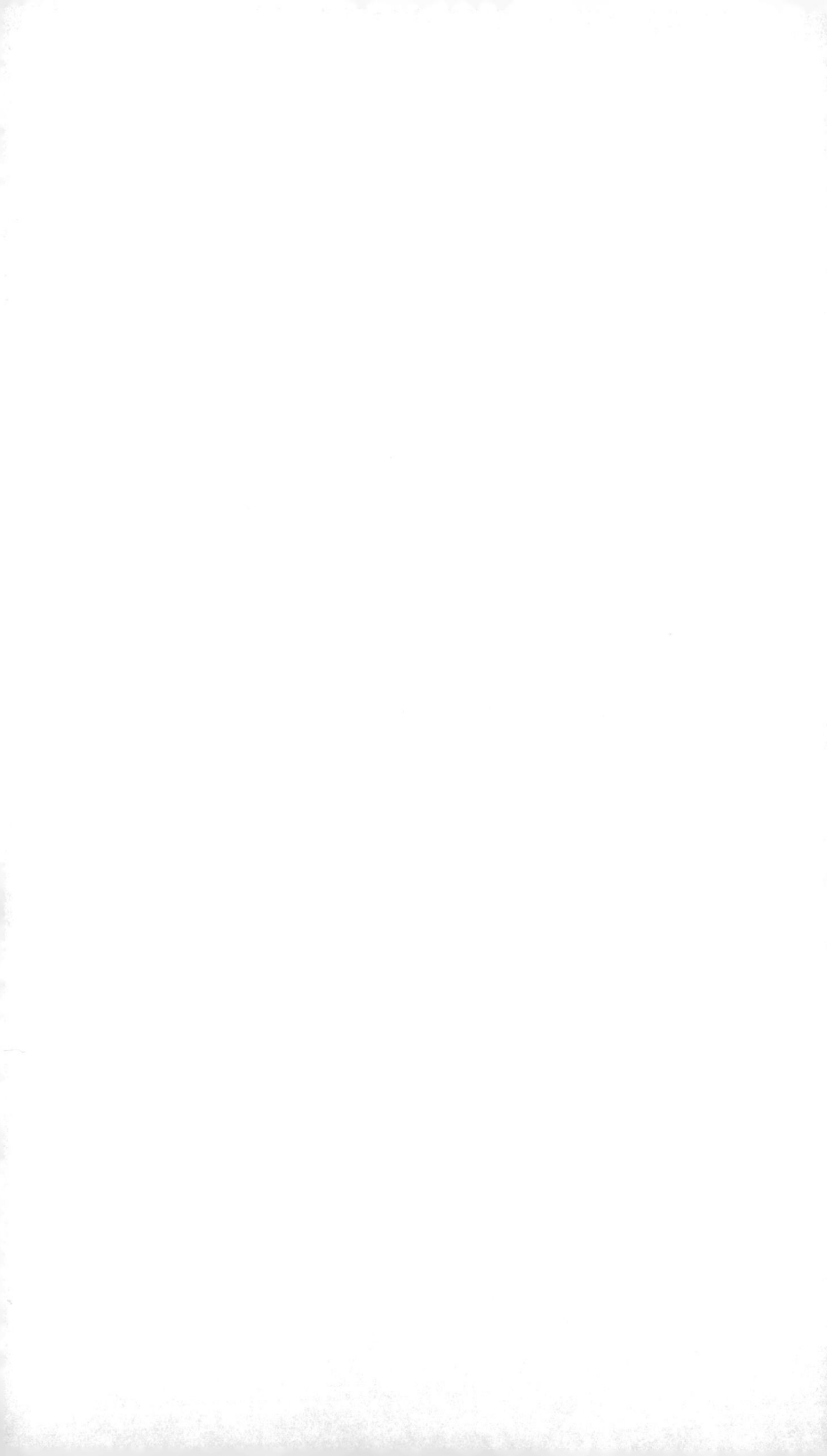

# Proper Care *and* Feeding Of Hemorrhoids

Lana Kay Murphy

To all my fellow sufferers

# ACKNOWLEDGEMENTS

Thanks to an unknown physician, who, like me, suffered from hemorrhoids. It was your pain that led you to writing a book that I needed to read. I found the book in 1985 and have searched diligently for it since with no luck. At the time I found it, it was stuffed randomly on a shelf obviously incorrectly placed because I wasn't even looking for something I very much needed. So, to whoever you are, my deepest thanks and appreciation for allowing the last 30 years to be mostly pain-free. And for anyone who has suffered the way I did, I pray this book may fall into your lap as serendipitously as the book I found did for me.

# Table of Contents

# Foreword

This section is included so that you can decide through the sample whether you even want to buy it. That's what samples are for, right?

First of all, I want you to know I'm a follower of Christ. I am grateful for a living God who loves us enough to have sent his son to atone for our sins. I believe Christ lived and died for us, that he paid the price for our sin so we don't have to, and that he died and was resurrected so all of us can have the gift of resurrection. We will all live again and have perfected bodies. Until then, we have imperfect bodies that were designed by God to heal themselves.

If you are in a lot of pain, I suggest you go soak in a tub of hot water and gently tuck your hemorrhoids where they belong. I know it sounds counter-intuitive to even touch something that is causing so much discomfort, but tucking your hemorrhoids inside really helps the pain. If you are still in agonizing pain after you have tucked in your hemorrhoids, you might have a more serious condition, and I would recommend talking to your doctor.

I first wrote this book in 2008 but set it aside because I'm not a physician. I have no credentials. How could I have anything valuable to say? However, I just suffered a severe episode after over thirty years of no problems. It happened after I had either a bad flu bug or food poisoning. I'm not sure which it was. The end result was my sitting on the toilet with a bucket in my lap having things come out at both ends. Not a pretty picture. It ended up with a flare up of hemorrhoids. I've been in that same scene before with no flare up, so I know I can get through the flu or food poisoning or pregnancy without having a problem. This time, I didn't, and I wondered what I had done different after all these years.

After puzzling about it, I realized what I had (or hadn't) done. Because I am in the middle of writing a novel, I hadn't been exercising the way I know I should. If exercise scares you, don't run yet. The exercise I'm talking about is a five-minute walk down the block and back. It's not aerobic. It's just moving. Sitting for hours at my desk typing with no movement was a bigger factor in my flare up than the stomach virus. Even though I was in the middle of a flare up and walking was painful, I forced myself to get back into a routine of walking. It's not a lot. Anyone can do it, and it makes a huge difference in your health.

So if you don't want to buy the book, take the time to move, eat fiber, tuck your hemorrhoids in, don't ever strain at the toilet, and don't ever have anal sex. Wait, what?? Yes, that last one. There are no sexual organs in or around the anus in either male or female human. There just aren't. Any pleasure doesn't come from the anus or the intestine. In fact, the lining of the intestine wasn't designed for friction. Any foreign object inside can tear the lining and cause a spreading of bacteria. It's not a healthy practice. A quick search on Google for hemorrhoids and you will find they are associated with anal sex. If the link is so clear that you find it with any search, you need to stop the practice right now. If you're not willing to do that, quit reading because this book won't help you.

# History

If you have no interest in history, you can skip to the next chapter.

For anyone who might like to know, hemorrhoids were mentioned as a plague in the Bible. In 1 Samuel 4-6, it talks about the Philistines and how they took the Ark of the Covenant from the Israelites. Chapter 5, verse 5 says "But the hand of the Lord was heavy upon them of Ashdod, and he destroyed them, and smote them with emerods, even Ashdod and the coasts thereof." It is mentioned again in Verse 9 in the same chapter. The Philistines moved the ark and the result? "The hand of the Lord was against the city with a very great destruction: and he smote the men of the city, both small and great, and they had emerods in their secret parts." So the Ark was moved again. Chapter 5, Verse 12 "And the men that died not were smitten with the emerods: and the cry of the city went up to heaven."

For anyone who has suffered from hemorrhoids, you can understand why the "cry of the city went up to heaven." If just the arrival of the Ark created such pain and discomfort, you'd want it gone, too.

I know none of us today have an Ark arriving in our city to create hemorrhoids, but some of us are living a lifestyle that is creating the problem. Anal sex is one of them. You can Google it. As I mentioned in the foreword, if you're doing it, stop.

According to a September 24, 1993, article about Napoleon, his loss at Waterloo was more about hemorrhoids than about his troops' abilities. You can read the article here: http://articles.chicagotribune.com/1993-09-24/news/9309240118_1_hemorrhoids-veins-pain

My own great-grandfather died from complications from hemorrhoid surgery. You have to be in a lot of pain to endure that kind of surgery. My husband's grandmother went through hemorrhoid surgery twice. She was telling me about it and said, "You could hear my screams down the hall when I had my first BM." You know she was hurting if she was willing to endure the pain of a bowel movement after surgery more than once. I understood her pain, but a non-surgical answer made more sense to me.

In our modern society where prostates and breasts are discussed openly in relation to the cancer that can take root in them, the discussion of a much more common ailment is somehow considered taboo.

How many people in today's modern era have died from hemorrhoids or its complications? We probably will never know. Unlike cancer, where a sufferer can be said to have fought a brave battle against it, the sufferers of hemorrhoids all suffer in embarrassed silence.

During the rarely-aired commercial for Preparation H, very little is said about the condition other than that instant relief can be obtained by using it. The only other mention might be in printed ads for the successful removal of hemorrhoidal tissue.

What these surgery ads never tell you is that it is very rare for a hemorrhoid sufferer to endure just one surgery for the condition. If the underlying problem is not understood, the sufferer will continue to act in a way designed to re-create the condition. It's like operating on lung cancer on a heavy smoker. The cancer might be removed, but the likelihood of its return is quite high because the patient is continuing the lifestyle that created the cancer in the first place.

I have been a lifelong sufferer of hemorrhoids. From the moment I was aware of my small body at the tender age of three, I had severe and constant problems with constipation and the pain of hemorrhoids. As I moved into the teen years, I could count on a monthly battle with painful piles. This generally occurred during my monthly cycle. The pain of piles accompanied by cramps made my cycle an almost unendurable week of pain.

As a young adult, I can remember several times where I could do nothing but curl into a fetal position on the floor just praying for my pain to stop. Only another hemorrhoid sufferer could relate to this kind of pain, and there are far too many sufferers out there, all feeling very much alone.

It was during one of these extremely painful episodes where I could hardly walk that I happened upon a small book in the basement of the library at Brigham Young University. I was researching another topic but stumbled upon this book on hemorrhoids. It changed my life.

It was written by a physician who was suffering from hemorrhoids and couldn't find a single book on the topic. I have searched since and haven't been able to find his book. All I know is that he was a medical doctor and the title of the book included something about hemorrhoids.

The book that saved my life is out of print. It was out of print when I found it. Written in the 1970s, I found it in the mid-1980s. I have searched for a similar book over the years and have never been able to find one. However, I did a search this week and found a few books on the topic. None of them have exactly the same information I have to share. I hope this booklet will add to the conversation.

I am going to share with you the overall ideas I found that helped me.

No cure will remove the scars that have developed. Even surgery will leave scarring. If you have as severe a case as I had, your scars will stay with you throughout your life. As you have noticed through the years, scars might look ugly but they don't hurt. Not one bit. And so my hemorrhoids have remained pretty much pain-free. Until this week, but it was a good reminder that I have something that needs to be shared.

Here are the steps to curing hemorrhoids:

Step one: Understand your body.
Step two: Eat fiber.
Step three: RELAX.
Step four: Be clean.
Step five: Exercise.
Step six: Pray.

These six simple steps can change your life. They changed mine.

I have given birth to three children without having my hemorrhoids flare up. Since I have diarrhea the whole pregnancy, any hemorrhoid sufferer would understand exactly what that means. It wasn't until I quit doing one of the basic steps (exercise) that I had a problem. If you follow these steps, you should be as pain free as I have been, and I'm planning to get back there by the end of the week. A flare up usually lasts three to seven days. Knowing there is an end in sight is a great relief.

# Understanding your body

O ur bodies are designed to perform their natural functions without pain (except, of course, in the case of child birth). Hemorrhoid sufferers wish that was true. How can something that should be easy—the elimination of body waste—turn into something so excruciatingly difficult and painful?

The answer lies in understanding how our bodies work.

Since this is the analogy that stuck with me, I am going to use the same one.

When a woman is expecting a baby, she can try to push that baby out through her whole pregnancy. Unless there is a physical problem with the cervix, no amount of pushing is going to get that baby out. The cervix has to be properly thinned and opened in a natural process, and this normally happens when the baby is physically ready to be delivered.

In the same way, the anus is designed to hold all of its contents until the proper time. If this wasn't the case, modern society would have to change the way everyone dressed. There'd be an awful lot of freak accidents happening at any given moment.

Fortunately, our bodies are designed to hold the waste until proper dumping time.

This design system is intricate, and much of it involves blood. As you know, our bodies are full of veins and arteries. The veins in the anus are large. They are designed to control the sphincter muscles.

When you relax at the time of defecation and your body is ready to release its contents, the blood leaves the area and the bowel movement can easily start. No pushing should happen when the bowel movement is first starting.

Pushing forces blood into the rectal area. This rush of blood narrows the passageway and makes the movement of the bowel very difficult. In essence, you are closing the hole that the feces needs to travel through.

After the bowel movement starts, pushing is just as necessary as when a woman is giving birth. However, pushing at the wrong moment is closing everything off. If you strain at the start, you are severely injuring your own body. You need to learn how to work with yourself.

If you are struggling with this concept, close your left fist tightly and then try to push your right pointer finger through. You could do it, but it would be difficult. That is what you are doing when you strain at the beginning of a bowel movement.

# Eat Fiber

Treat white bread like excrement. It is. Hard.

If you're a woman who has had a baby in a hospital, you have probably noticed the hospital diets. White bread, milk, pudding, cooked vegetables, meat. The only item on the menu with fiber is a little fruit. No wonder so many women have hemorrhoids!

Switch to high-fiber pastas and cereals. Sprinkle bran, chia seeds, teff seeds or flax seeds on your yogurt. The seeds are an excellent source of fiber and essential fatty acids.

If you can't seem to get enough fiber in your diet, use a fiber supplement like Metamucil or Benefiber.

Fortunately, the benefits of fiber are well known now. It wasn't so much thirty years ago when I made my life-altering switch.

I recommend reading FIT FOR LIFE by Harvey and Marilyn Diamond. If you read the book and only change one thing, eat all your fruit first. Never serve raw fruit for dessert. Serve it as a palate cleanser. The fiber from the fruit will help the rest of the meal move through your body. The fruit also cleanses as it goes.

# RELAX

Get every written piece of material out of your bathroom. It is not a library. It is not a reading room. Take out those magazine stands. The newspaper should not go through the bathroom door.

This one item is probably the hardest to learn. If you have strained your whole life like I used to, relaxing seems like a totally foreign concept. It takes time and patience, but I promise, it does work.

If you feel the urge to go, walk quickly to the nearest bathroom. This is very important.

We have learned our whole lives to put off the urge. Don't.

I don't care if you're in an important meeting. They can wait five minutes.

If you're the teacher, call for a break.

Unless you're fighting a fire and someone's life is on the line, YOUR life is on the line. Get to the bathroom.

When you're on the toilet, relax. Wait 60 seconds. If nothing happens, get up and go about your duties. Walk around. Don't sit somewhere. Do something active. Do the dishes if you're at home or wash out the sink. If you're at work, walk to the water fountain. Walk to get a snack. Make it a high fiber one. Bananas are great.

DO NOT spend more than 60 seconds on the toilet waiting for a bowel movement to come. Get one of those sand timers meant for timing tooth brushing. When the sand runs out, GET OFF the toilet.

You will NEVER cure your hemorrhoids if you do not learn this step.

So, you feel the urge, GO to the bathroom. RELAX for 60 seconds. If nothing happens, get up and do something else. When the urge happens again, sit down and time yourself again.

When you are first learning how to relax, it might take several times before a bowel movement will start. Don't worry. It will happen.

At this point, I do want to make a cautionary statement. Bowel obstructions are real and can be deadly. If you are in extreme pain, please see a doctor. Immediately seek medical attention for any pain that seems abnormal.

The above steps can seem especially difficult if you are having diarrhea. However, you *can* relax through the process. When you feel done, get up and walk around. If you feel the urge to go, sit down and relax again. Sitting and straining even if your gut feels like it is going to explode will only put you in pain. I know. I've been there.

Relax. It works.

The other item I wanted to discuss under relaxation is gas.

I was raised to be a lady. Ladies simply do not pass gas. It's unthinkable. Any embarrassing odor or sound is to be avoided at all cost.

Unfortunately, denying your body's natural function of dispelling gas not only causes very painful stomach aches but is also a factor in hemorrhoids.

I am not saying that you should embarrass your friends and co-workers by a thoughtless, uncaring attitude about gas. I'm a mom, and I still ask my children for some decorum.

However, holding in gas is a physical problem. You can leave the room, go to the bathroom, make some effort to be by yourself, but don't hold in the gas. Do whatever you need to do, but don't hold it in. Hemorrhoids are a sure result.

So relax on the toilet. Count to 60. And don't hold in the gas (but please be polite).

# Be Clean

Unless you can't stand the thought of spending money on wipe ups, I recommend that you keep some moist wipes in every bathroom in your house. Keep a stash on hand at work. If you can't stand the thought of spending the money, then you need to get your toilet paper moist. Flush the toilet and use clean water.

Whichever way you do it, make sure you end your bathroom session with a moist cleansing. This gets all the feces off your bottom. If you aren't clean, you will feel the urge to go before your body is actually ready to defecate.

When you are in the middle of a hemorrhoid attack, take several hot soaking baths a day. The hot water can help ease the pain. At the time of your bath, tuck the painful hemorrhoids into your rectum. The pressure from your sphincter will help reduce the pressure of the blood in the tissue, which reduces the pain.

If you're at work and can't take a bath, squeeze your sphincter muscles and count to 10, then relax. When the pain is intense, putting pressure on the veins does help ease it.

Remember that even a very painful episode usually won't last more than a week. If it does, you will want to talk to your doctor about having a colonoscopy or other examination for cancer. Recent studies have shown that MRIs can detect suspicious polyps in the colon, so a less-invasive procedure might be better for you. Hemorrhoids make the invasive procedures almost unthinkable. Discuss the options with your doctor.

Remember to moist clean after a bowel movement, and soak in the tub whenever you're having an episode.

# Exercise

I know. You hear it every day. Exercise. It helps your heart. It helps you lose weight. It helps you live longer. It also helps with your hemorrhoids, so do it.

I am one of those people that has to be forced to exercise. At one point, I got a job scrubbing floors from 6 to 8 am four days a week. I would never get out of bed at 5:30 am to exercise, but I will get out of bed for a job. If that's what it takes to get you moving, get a job.

I'm currently working at a sitting job, so I get my exercise during my two fifteen-minute breaks. I walk around the parking lot or down the block and back. The walk takes about ten minutes twice a day. It's not strenuous, but as long as I'm faithful about it, I avoid flare ups. My most recent problem was a good reminder to stay active.

As you noticed in my relaxation section, walking when you can't start a bowel movement is a good way to get a bowel movement to start, or at least get your mind off your bowel movement when it won't start.

Exercise. It's good for your heart and your bowels.

# Pray

This actually should be step one. It was the first step I took, and my guess is if you are reading this booklet, it was your first step also.

There is a God in Heaven that hears and answers prayers. He knows you. He knows your pain, and he desires to heal you. Mathew 7:7-8 reminds us "Ask, and it shall be given you; seek, and ye shall find; knock, and it shall be opened unto you: For every one that asketh receiveth; and he that seeketh findeth; and to him that knocketh it shall be opened."

You can heal. God can help. Ask for his assistance in your life. You will find the answers you need.

# Do It

You now know the steps for healing hemorrhoids. They are simple, and they can change your life. They have changed mine. I will forever bear the scars, but I have been pain free, and you can be, too. Start today.

RELAX.

You can do this, and God will help you.

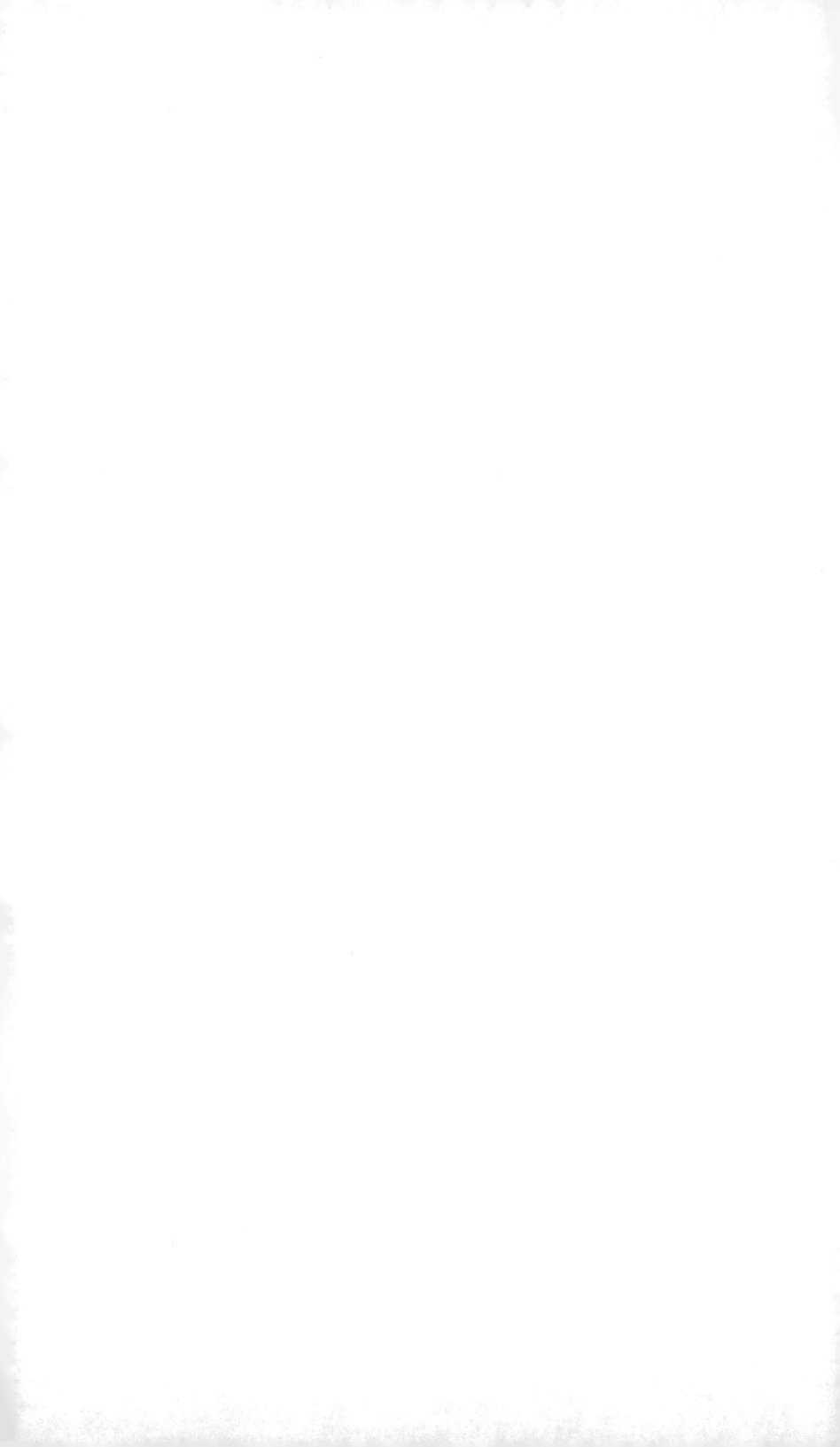